DIET OF THE MEDITERRANEAN BOOK:

A detailed diet book for ages

By

Crystal M. Thompson

DISCLAIMER PAGE

Table of Content

INTRODUCTION

The Mediterranean Diet places a premium on plant-based meals and healthy fats. You consume a lot of vegetables, fruits, and whole grains. The major source of fat is olive oil. According to research, the Mediterranean Diet may reduce your risk of cardiovascular disease and a variety of other chronic illnesses. A dietician may assist you in tailoring the diet to your specific requirements.

What exactly is the Mediterranean Diet?

The Mediterranean Diet is an eating plan that focuses on plant-based meals and healthy fats.

In general, a Mediterranean Diet consists of the following foods:

- Vegetables, fruits, beans, lentils, and nuts in plenty.
- Whole grains, such as whole-wheat bread and brown rice, are abundant.
- Plenty of extra virgin olive oil (EVOO) as a healthy fat source.
- A modest quantity of fish, particularly omega-3 fatty acid-rich seafood.
- A healthy serving of cheese and yogurt.
- Little or no meat, preferring chicken over red meat.
- There should be no sweets, sugary drinks, or butter.

A reasonable quantity of wine with meals (but don't start if you don't already).Based on your medical history, underlying diseases, allergies, and preferences, a nutritionist may help you alter your diet as required.

CHAPTER 1

What does the Mediterranean Diet entail?

There are several definitions of the diet (each with somewhat different serving objectives). This is because the diet emphasizes general eating habits over specific formulae or computations. It's also based on eating habits in a variety of Mediterranean nations, each with its unique quirks. Because there is no standard definition, the Mediterranean Diet is adaptable and may be tailored to your specific requirements.

What are the advantages of a Mediterranean diet?

The Mediterranean Diet offers several advantages, including:

- Lowering your chances of developing cardiovascular disease.
- Helping you maintain a healthy body weight.
- Helping to maintain appropriate blood sugar, blood pressure, and cholesterol levels.
- Lowering your chances of developing metabolic syndrome.
- Aiding in the maintenance of a healthy balance of gut microbiota (bacteria and other microbes) in your digestive tract.
- Lowering your chances of developing certain forms of cancer.
- Slowing the deterioration of brain function as you become older.

The Mediterranean Diet is often recommended by cardiologists because significant evidence supports its heart-healthy effects. Over five years, one research (published in 2018) looked at patients at high risk of cardiovascular disease. The Mediterranean Diet was followed by one group, whereas the low-fat diet was followed by the other. When compared to the low-fat diet group, the

Mediterranean Diet group had a 30% reduced relative risk of cardiovascular events.

Researchers think that the Mediterranean Diet's healthy fats contribute to these preventive advantages. These are derived from foods such as olive oil, almonds, and seafood.

Why is the Mediterranean Diet beneficial to me?

The Mediterranean Diet has a variety of nutrients that work together to benefit your health. There is no one item or ingredient that is responsible for the advantages of the Mediterranean Diet. Instead, the diet is beneficial due to the mix of nutrients it supplies.

Consider a choir with numerous members singing. One voice may carry part of the music, but all voices must work together to get the entire impact. Similarly, the Mediterranean Diet works by providing you with a perfect combination of nutrients that work together to maintain your health.

A Mediterranean diet is beneficial since it:

- Reduces saturated and trans fats. Saturated fat is necessary, but only in modest quantities. Saturated fat consumption may increase LDL (bad) cholesterol. A high LDL level increases the risk of artery plaque development (atherosclerosis). There are no health advantages to eating trans fat. Both of these "unhealthy fats" have the potential to produce inflammation.
- Encourages the consumption of healthful unsaturated fats, such as omega-3 fatty acids. Unsaturated fats improve good cholesterol levels, brain function,

and inflammation reduction. Furthermore, eating a diet rich in unsaturated fats and low in saturated fat supports good blood sugar levels.

- Limits sodium intake. A high-sodium diet may elevate your blood pressure, increasing your risk of a heart attack or stroke.
- Refined carbs, especially sugar, are restricted. Refined carbohydrate foods may trigger blood sugar spikes. Refined carbohydrates can provide more calories with no nutritional value. Such foods, for example, often have little or no fiber.
- Foods rich in fiber and antioxidants are preferred. These nutrients aid in the reduction of inflammation throughout the body. Fiber also aids in the movement of waste through your big intestine. Antioxidants defend against cancer by combating free radicals.

What exactly is the Mediterranean Diet?

The Mediterranean Diet looks different for everyone. It contains a lot of whole grains, vegetables, and fruit, as well as modest portions of fish, legumes, and nuts.

Dietitians often propose the serving goals and advice shown in the chart below. It's important to speak with a dietician about your specific requirements and objectives so that you may create the best plan for you.

Food	Serving Objective	Size of a Serving	Tips
Fruits and vegetables that are in season.	3 servings of fruit per day; 3 servings of vegetables per day.	12 cups to 1 cup fruit; 12 cups cooked or 1 cup raw vegetables.	Consume at least one serving of vegetables at each meal and fruit as a snack.
Starchy veggies (potatoes, peas, and maize) and whole grains.	Three to six servings each day.	12 cups cooked grains, pasta, or cereal; 1 slice bread; 1 cup dry cereal.	Bake or roast red-skinned potatoes or sweet potatoes; choose whole grain bread, cereal, couscous, and pasta; limit or eliminate processed carbs.
EVOO (extra virgin olive oil).	1-2 servings each day.	1 tsp.	Use vegetable oil and animal fats (butter, sourcream, mayo);drizzle over salads,cooked vegetables,or pasta; dip bread in.
Beans and lentils	Three servings	½ cup.	Add to salads,

are legumes.	every week.		soups, and pasta meals; serve with raw vegetables in hummus or bean dip; or choose a veggie or bean burger.
Fish.	Three servings every week.	3.5 to 4 oz.	Choose omega-3-rich seafood such as salmon, sardines, herring, tuna, and mackerel.
Nuts.	At least three times every week	¼ cup nuts or 2 tablespoons nut butter.	Select walnuts, almonds, and hazelnuts as a snack; add to cereal, salad, and yogurt; select raw, unsalted, and dry roasted kinds; and eat alone or with dried fruit.

Poultry.	No more than once each day (less is best).	Three ounces.	Use white meat over dark meat; substitute red meat for white meat; use skinless fowl or remove the skin before cooking; bake, broil, or grill it.
Dairy.	No more than once each day (less is best).	1 cup milk or yogurt; 1 ½ ounces natural cheese.	Choose naturally low-fat cheese; fat-free or 1% milk, yogurt, and cottage cheese; and avoid whole-fat milk, cream, and sauces and dressings made with cream.
Eggs.	1 yolk per day is allowed.	1 whole egg (yolk and white).	restriction on egg yolks; no restriction on egg whites; no more than four yolks per

			week if you have excessive cholesterol.
Beef, hog, veal, and lamb are examples of red meat.	No more than one serving each week.	Three ounces.	Limit yourself to thin cuts like tenderloin, sirloin, and flank steak.
Desserts and baked products.	Limit handmade items to no more than three servings per week; avoid commercially produced baked goods and sweets.	Depending on the kind.	Instead, use fruit and nonfat yogurt; bake with liquid oil rather than solid fats; whole grain flour rather than bleached or enhanced flour; and egg whites rather than entire eggs.
Wine is optional.	1 serving per day (for persons born female); 2 servings per day	1 glass.	If you don't drink, the American Heart Association advises you not to

	(for people born male).		start; instead, consult with your healthcare physician about the advantages and hazards of drinking in moderation.

CHAPTER 2

How can I begin the Mediterranean Diet?

- As you begin a new eating plan, you may have numerous questions. Before making dramatic dietary changes or attempting any new eating plan, talk with your primary care physician or a dietician. They will ensure that your planned strategy is ideal for you based on your specific demands. They'll also send you meal ideas and recipes to try at home.

- As you begin, you may worry about how much you can change about the Mediterranean Diet without losing its advantages. Remember that the Mediterranean Diet is a general dietary plan. It is not a rigorous diet with stringent regulations. As a consequence, you may tailor it to your specific requirements (preferably with the assistance of a dietician).

The following are answers to some often-asked questions concerning alterations:

- Can the Mediterranean Diet be followed by vegetarians?

Yes. If you want a vegetarian diet, the Mediterranean Diet may be readily modified to omit meat and fish. In such a situation, your protein would come entirely from plant sources such as nuts and beans. To learn more, speak with a dietician.

- Is it possible to follow a gluten-free Mediterranean diet?

Yes. You may adapt recipes to omit gluten-containing ingredients. Consult a dietician for recipe ideas and assistance in making the required modifications.

- Can I use normal olive oil with extra virgin olive oil?

Regular olive oil is a healthy option for high-saturated-fat oils like palm oil. However, extra virgin olive oil provides the highest advantages.

Before embarking on the Mediterranean Diet, it is critical to understand that not all olive oils are created equal. The Mediterranean Diet especially recommends extra virgin olive oil (EVOO). This is due to its healthy fat ratio. This indicates that EVOO includes more good (unsaturated) fat than harmful (saturated) fat. Aside from its fat ratio, EVOO is healthful due to its strong antioxidant content. Antioxidants aid in the protection of your heart and the reduction of inflammation throughout your body. Regular olive oil does not contain these antioxidants since it is made differently.

- Can I eat pizza while following the Mediterranean Diet?

It is dependent on how you cook it. The salt, saturated fat, and calories in many American-style pizzas are excessive. These factors make it less than optimal for achieving your Mediterranean Diet objectives. To gain greater nutritional advantages, make your own heart-healthy pizza instead of ordering out.

- Can I consume cuisine from civilizations other than the Mediterranean?

The Mediterranean Diet outlines eating habits in one region of the globe. That doesn't imply you should avoid dishes and recipes from different cultures.

It is important to create an eating plan that is good for you physically, mentally, and socially. The Mediterranean Diet is a manner of eating that has been linked to several health advantages by study. This diet focuses on typical eating behaviors. It does not need you to study every single dietary decision or to avoid certain foods.

As a result, the Mediterranean Diet may be tailored to your interests and cultural customs. This might imply sticking to classic dishes (no ingredient replacements) and only eating them on rare occasions. Some recipes may be just as wonderful and unique to you if you use olive oil instead of butter or additional herbs instead of salt. Working with a dietician may assist you in determining when and how to make replacements or other adjustments to your significant recipes.

What is the relationship between lifestyle and the Mediterranean Diet?

To get the most out of your diet, strive to:

- Exercise on a regular basis, preferably with others.
- Cook and share meals with family and friends.
- You should cook more frequently than you eat out.
- When possible, eat foods obtained locally.
- When did the Mediterranean Diet come into being? The Mediterranean Diet was first proposed in the 1950s.

So, if you eat the Mediterranean Diet now, you're eating as people in specific Mediterranean nations did in the mid-20th century. According to research, such trends have evolved over time and are no longer valid in many Mediterranean nations.

There are visual pyramids and other instructions that demonstrate how to follow a Mediterranean Diet. A dietitian can assist you in reviewing such materials and explaining how to utilize them in your everyday life.

It might be difficult to decide which diet is best for you in a world where there are so many possibilities. The Mediterranean Diet has been shown in studies to benefit many individuals, particularly those at risk of heart disease.

Aside from heart health, the Mediterranean Diet may help you avoid or treat a variety of other ailments.

Before embarking on any dietary regimen, it is critical to consult with a healthcare expert. They will ensure that the plan is suitable for you and will assist you in making any necessary changes. Inform your loved ones about your aspirations as well. Invite them to prepare and dine with you. When you have a supportive group to help you along the road, it is simpler to stick to an eating plan over time.

CHAPTER 3

Foods to consume and foods to avoid

The Mediterranean diet emphasizes plant foods more than many other diets. Fruits, vegetables, whole grains, and legumes are common components of meals and snacks. Small servings of fish, pork, or eggs may be included in meals. For taste, people often cook with olive oil and add herbs and spices.

Foods

The following foods are prioritized in a Mediterranean-style eating pattern Source:

- a wide range of fresh fruits and veggies
- complete grains
- legumes
- Olive oil, nuts, seeds, and fatty seafood are all good sources of healthy fats.
- modest seafood consumption
- low dairy and red meat consumption
- While moderate quantities of red wine are suitable for meals, water and sugar-free drinks, such as sparkling water and fresh juices, may help individuals keep hydrated.

Snacks

When following a Mediterranean diet, aim to choose snacks packed with nutritional components. Here are several possibilities:

- fresh fruit and a handful of nuts
- Greek yogurt, unsweetened, topped with fresh fruit and sunflower nuts
- Hummus and seasonal veggies
- Trail mix prepared from nuts and dried fruit that hasn't been sweetened

- roasted chickpeas with herbs
- berries and cottage cheese
- a hard-boiled egg with some cheese and some fresh fruit

Meal plan for 7 days

Here's an example of a Mediterranean diet food plan for 7 days:

Day 1: Breakfast Frittata of vegetables and eggs served with sliced avocado over whole grain bread

Add another egg for more calories.

A huge green salad with a baked salmon fillet, red onion, feta cheese, quinoa, and fresh tomatoes for lunch

Pita bread made with whole grains

hummus (two ounces)

Spicy lentil soup with spinach for dinner

Day 2: For breakfast, make a Greek yogurt parfait with walnuts, fresh berries, and chia seeds.

Add 1-2 ounces of almonds for added calories.

Greek chicken grain bowls for lunch with olives, cucumbers, and red onions

Add hummus or avocado to increase the calorie count.

Baked fish with garlic roasted potatoes and asparagus for dinner

Day 3: Breakfast Steel-cut or rolled oats with fresh fruit, sliced almonds or almond butter, and honey drizzle.

Salad with chickpeas and farro for lunch

Dinner Mediterranean shrimp with whole-wheat pasta

Day 4: Shakshuka, a meal of poached eggs in a sauce of tomatoes, olive oil, peppers, onion, and garlic that is frequently seasoned with cumin, paprika, and cayenne pepper.

Large green salad with fresh veggies, lentils, sunflower seeds, and grilled shrimp for lunch

Roasted chicken with roasted root vegetables and Brussels sprouts for dinner

Day 5: Breakfast Poached egg on top of sweet potato breakfast hash

Lentil and tuna salad for lunch

Mediterranean spaghetti for dinner

Day 6: Chia pudding with fresh berries and almond butter for breakfast.

Lunch consists of a Mediterranean white bean soup and a Greek salad.

Dinner Baked fish with garlic and basil served with quinoa salad caprese

Day 7: Overnight oats with nut butter and berries for breakfast

Mediterranean Buddha bowl for lunch

Balsamic roasted chicken and veggies for dinner

Health Advantages

The following are some of the possible advantages of a Mediterranean diet.

- Reduced risk of cardiovascular disease: A Mediterranean diet may lessen the risk of cardiovascular events in those who already have heart disease, according to research. For almost 5 years, one research compared two Mediterranean diets against a control diet. According to the study, the diet lowered the risk of cardiovascular disorders such as stroke, heart attack, and mortality by roughly 30% when compared to the control group.
More research is required to understand if lifestyle variables such as physical activity and wider social support networks contribute to the lower prevalence of heart disease in Mediterranean nations compared to the United States.

- Enhancing Sleep Quality: Researchers investigated how the Mediterranean diet impacts sleep in a 2018 studyTrusted Source.According to their findings, following a Mediterranean diet may enhance sleep quality in older persons. In younger persons, the diet had no effect on sleep quality.

- Weight reduction:The Mediterranean diet may aid with weight management.

Summary

A Mediterranean diet may be recommended by doctors to help prevent illness and keep individuals healthy for a longer period of time. Because the Mediterranean area offers a diverse range of foods and cuisines, there is no unique Mediterranean diet, but rather a way of eating.

A dietician may assist a person in developing a meal plan that is tailored to their specific requirements and the foods at their disposal. Because not everyone in the Mediterranean area eats the same way, the Mediterranean dietary pattern is intended to be a flexible guidance for a balanced and diverse diet that favors plant-based foods.

Commonly Asked Questions

Here are some frequently asked questions concerning the Mediterranean diet.

What precisely does a Mediterranean diet entail?

There is no such thing as a Mediterranean diet. Rather, it is a way of eating that emphasizes fresh, unprocessed meals, a wide range of fruits and vegetables, and whole foods. Protein is found in seafood, fish, dairy products, and lentils, as well as some meat.

What are the top ten Mediterranean diet foods?

The following are ten food categories that are likely to appear in a Mediterranean diet:

vegetables

fruits

beans

lentils

nuts

complete grains

fish

seafood

Extra virgin olive oil

yogurt

What does a typical Mediterranean breakfast consist of?

This can vary depending on where you are in the Mediterranean, but some alternatives include:

olive oil on whole wheat bread

fruit

unprocessed cheeses such as ricotta, feta, cottage, and others

olives

fruit juice, freshly squeezed

Tomato and peppers with eggs

Is it possible to consume potatoes on a Mediterranean diet?

Potatoes are vegetables that may be used in a variety of Mediterranean cuisines, such as this Greek potato salad with lemon, garlic, and parsley.

Ready-made fries, on the other hand, are not part of a Mediterranean diet. The taste should originate from the potato itself, rather than from salt, garnishes, or heavily processed additives or flavorings.

Summary

Making long-term, sustainable food decisions is part of following a Mediterranean diet.

In general, a person should strive for a diet rich in natural foods, such as lots of veggies, whole grains, and healthy fats.

Anyone who does not feel satisfied with their food should see a dietician. They might suggest extra or different meals to assist in promoting fullness.

A guide to eating a healthy diet
It consists of meals from five dietary categories, including veggies, protein, and whole grains, and may aid with weight management and illness prevention.

Dietary standards change in response to scientific breakthroughs, making it difficult to keep current and know what to consume.

In this post, we will examine current dietary guidelines and explain how to create a balanced diet.

A balanced diet is one that meets all of a person's nutritional requirements. Humans need a specific number of calories and nutrients to maintain their health.

A balanced diet includes all of the nutrients a person needs while staying under the daily calorie limit.

People may receive the nutrients and calories they need by eating a balanced diet and avoiding junk food or food with little nutritional value.

Following a dietary pyramid was formerly recommended by the United States Department of Agriculture (USDA). However, as nutritional knowledge has progressed, they now advocate consuming items from each of the five food categories and constructing a balanced plate.

According to USDA guidelines, half of a person's plate should be made up of fruits and vegetables.

The remaining half should be composed of grains and protein. They suggest having a dish of low-fat dairy or another source of the nutrients present in dairy with each meal.

The five food categories

A healthy, well-balanced diet comprises items from the following five categories:

vegetables

fruits

grains

protein

dairy

Vegetables

The vegetable category is divided into five subgroups:

greens with leaves

veggies that are crimson or orange

veggies with a high starch content

legumes (beans and peas)

Additional veggies like eggplant and zucchini

People should eat a variety of veggies to receive essential nutrients and avoid dietary monotony.

Furthermore, the USDA recommends that consumers eat vegetables from each of the five groupings at least once a week.

Vegetables may be eaten raw or prepared. It is crucial to note, however, that boiling vegetables destroys part of their nutritious content. Furthermore, certain procedures, such as deep-frying, might introduce unhealthy fats into a meal.

Fruits

Fruit is an important part of a well-balanced diet. Instead of drinking juice, nutritionists urge eating entire fruits.

Juice is deficient in nutrients. Furthermore, the production process often adds useless calories owing to additional sugar. Instead of syrup, people should eat fresh or frozen fruits, or fruits canned in water.

Grains

Whole grains and processed grains are the two subcategories.

Whole grains include all three sections of the grain: bran, germ, and endosperm. Because whole grains are broken down slowly by the body, they have less of an impact on blood sugar levels.

Furthermore, whole grains include more fiber and protein than processed grains.

Refined grains have been treated and lack the three original components. Refined grains are also lower in protein and fiber and can cause blood sugar spikes.

Grains used to be at the bottom of the government-approved food pyramid, which meant that grains accounted for the majority of a person's daily caloric intake.

However, according to the updated guidelines, grains should account for only one-quarter of a person's plate.

Whole grains should account for at least half of a person's daily grain intake. Whole grains that are good for you include:

- quinoa
- oats
- rice (brown)
- barley
- buckwheat
- Protein

According to the 2015-2020 Dietary Guidelines for Americans, all persons should incorporate nutrient-dense protein in their daily diet.

According to the recommendations, this protein should account for one-quarter of a person's plate.

Proteins that are high in nutrients include:

- beef and pork that is lean
- turkey and chicken
- fish
- legumes, peas, and beans

Dairy

Calcium is found in dairy and fortified soy products. When feasible, the USDA recommends eating low-fat alternatives.

Low-fat dairy and soy products include the following:

- cottage cheese or ricotta
- milk with a reduced fat content
- yogurt
- soybean milk
- Lactose intolerant people may select low-lactose or lactose-free products, or soy-based calcium and other nutritional sources.

Weight loss

A poor diet is a frequent cause of weight loss difficulties.

A balanced diet, when paired with a regular exercise plan, may assist a person in lowering their risk factors for obesity or weight gain.

A well-balanced diet may aid in weight loss by:

- boosting their protein consumption
- Limiting your intake of carbs and processed meals
- obtaining important nutrients such as minerals, vitamins, and fiber
- avoiding binge eating
- People interested in decreasing weight should establish or strengthen their exercise program.

For some individuals, adding 30 minutes of walking each day and making simple modifications, such as using the stairs, might help them burn calories and lose weight.

For those who can, incorporating a moderate activity that incorporates cardio and strength training can assist in expediting weight reduction.

Summary

Consuming a balanced diet entails consuming foods from the five main groupings.

Dietary recommendations vary throughout time, as scientists find new facts about nutrition. Current guidelines say that a person's plate should comprise largely vegetables and fruits, some lean protein, some dairy, and soluble fiber.

People interested in weight reduction can also consider integrating moderate exercise into their habits.

CHAPTER 4

What is the best diet for osteoarthritis?

Changes to a person's diet may assist them to manage osteoarthritis symptoms. Eating specific foods and avoiding or restricting others may assist with controlling inflammation linked with arthritis, decreasing cholesterol, and more.

Osteoarthritis is the most prevalent type of arthritis, affecting nearly 30 million adultsTrusted Source in the United States. It arises when the cartilage in the joints breaks away over time.

The illness may affect any joint in the body, but patients typically experience pain in their knees, wrists, hips, or spine.

This book will discuss which foods persons with osteoarthritis should eat and which they should avoid. We also debunk some prevalent dietary fallacies about arthritis.

How might food aid in the treatment of osteoarthritis?

Specific foods or nutritional supplements cannot heal osteoarthritis, but some diets help alleviate symptoms, according to the Arthritis Foundation.

Some foods contain anti-inflammatory properties that may help lessen symptoms, while others might exacerbate them.

The proper diet may aid in the treatment of osteoarthritis in the following ways:

- Inflammation control and damage prevention

A well-balanced, healthy diet will provide the body with the tools it needs to avoid additional joint damage, which is critical for persons with osteoarthritis.

Some foods are known to lower inflammation in the body, and adhering to an anti-inflammatory diet may help alleviate symptoms. Consuming adequate antioxidants, such as vitamins A, C, and E, may assist in avoiding additional joint injury.

- Lowering cholesterol

People with osteoarthritis are more likely to have high blood cholesterol levels, and lowering cholesterol levels may alleviate the symptoms of this condition. People with the appropriate diet may swiftly improve their cholesterol levels.

- Keeping a healthy weight

Being overweight may put additional strain on the joints, and having too much fat in the body can create further inflammation. Maintaining a healthy weight might help to alleviate osteoarthritis symptoms.

Maintaining a healthy weight may be challenging for some individuals, particularly those who have a medical condition that limits their movement, such as osteoarthritis. A doctor or a dietician will be able to help.

Why should you consume these eight foods?

Specific nutrients may assist the body in battling inflammation and illness by strengthening the bones, muscles, and joints.

To alleviate symptoms of osteoarthritis, consider include the following eight items in your diet:

1. fatty fish

Omega-3 fatty acids are abundant in oily seafood. Because polyunsaturated fats have anti-inflammatory effects, they may be beneficial to patients suffering from osteoarthritis.

People suffering from osteoarthritis should consume at least one serving of oily salmon every week. Among the oily fish are:

- sardines
- mackerel
- salmon
- Tuna from the sea

Those who prefer not to consume fish may replace it with omega-3 supplements such as fish oil, krill oil, or flaxseed oil.

Trusted Source Chia seeds, flaxseed oil, and walnuts are other good sources of omega-3. These meals may also aid in the reduction of inflammation.

2. Oils

Other oils, in addition to oily fish, may help to decrease inflammation. Extra virgin olive oil includes a high concentration of oleocanthal, which has effects comparable to nonsteroidal anti-inflammatory medications (NSAIDs).

Avocado and safflower oils are both nutritious and may help decrease cholesterol.

3. Dairy

Calcium and vitamin D are abundant in milk, yogurt, and cheese. These nutrients strengthen bones, which may alleviate painful symptoms.

Dairy also includes proteins that may aid in muscle development. People who want to lose weight might choose low-fat choices.

4. Greens with dark leaves

Dark leafy greens are high in vitamin D as well as anti-stress phytochemicals and antioxidants. Vitamin D is required for calcium absorption and may stimulate the immune system, assisting the body in fighting illness.

Dark leafy greens include the following:

- spinach
- kale
- chard
- chard greens

5. Broccoli

Broccoli includes sulforaphane, a chemical that experts think may decrease the onset of osteoarthritis.

This crop is also high in vitamins K and C, as well as calcium, which helps to build bones.

6. Grass tea

Polyphenols are antioxidants that may be able to alleviate inflammation and delay the pace of cartilage deterioration, according to scientists. Polyphenols are abundant in green tea.

7. Garlic

Scientists think that a chemical found in garlic called diallyl disulfide may function against the enzymes in the body that destroy cartilage.

8. Nuts

Nuts are heart-healthy because they are abundant in calcium, magnesium, zinc, vitamin E, and fiber. They also include alpha-linolenic acid (ALA), which aids in immune system function.

What about the Mediterranean way of life?

According to research, the Mediterranean diet may help lower the inflammation that causes osteoarthritis symptoms.

A Mediterranean-style diet has many additional health advantages, including weight reduction, in addition to helping to alleviate the pain associated with osteoarthritis.

A Mediterranean diet may also lower your chances of:

- Stroke and heart disease
- muscle wasting in elderly age
- Alzheimer's disease is a neurological disorder.
- untimely death
- Fruits and vegetables, whole grains, legumes, seafood, yogurt, and healthy fats like olive oil and nuts are all part of the diet.

People may make easy dietary modifications to mimic the Mediterranean diet. These might include:

- consuming high-fiber, starchy foods like sweet potatoes, potatoes, beans, lentils, whole-grain bread and pasta
- consuming an abundance of fruits and veggies
- including seafood into the diet
- consuming less meat
- selecting items containing vegetable and plant oils, such as olive oil
- Choosing wholemeal alternatives over refined flour options
- Three foods to avoid, and why
- When a person has osteoarthritis, their body is in an inflammatory condition.

While anti-inflammatory meals may alleviate symptoms, certain foods include ingredients that actively promote inflammation. It is advised to avoid or limit certain food options.

Foods to avoid include those that include the following ingredients:

1. Sugar

Sugars that have been processed may cause the release of cytokines, which serve as inflammatory messengers in the body. Sugars added to sweetened beverages, such as soda, sweet tea, flavored coffees, and certain juice drinks, are the most likely to aggravate inflammatory diseases.

2. Saturated fatty acid

Saturated fat-rich foods, such as pizza and red meat, may trigger inflammation in the fat tissue. This may aggravate arthritic inflammation while also increasing the risk of obesity, heart disease, and other illnesses.

3. Carbohydrates that have been refined

Refined carbohydrates, such as white bread, white rice, and potato chips, promote the development of AGE oxidants. These have the potential to cause inflammation in the body.

CHAPTER 5

Three arthritis food misconceptions debunked

Many individuals believe that particular foods might aggravate osteoarthritis, but there isn't necessarily scientific proof to back up these claims.

Three popular misconceptions are discussed below:

1. Citrus fruits are inflammatory.

Some individuals feel that citrus fruits should be avoided because their acidity is inflammatory. This, however, is not the case. Citrus fruits, in fact, have anti-inflammatory properties in addition to being high in vitamin C and antioxidants.

Grapefruit juice, on the other hand, may interfere with several arthritis medications. Patients receiving treatment should consult with their doctor before introducing it into their diet.

2. Dairy avoidance aids in the treatment of osteoarthritis.

There is also evidence that eliminating dairy products may assist with osteoarthritis. Although milk, cheese, and other dairy products might be harmful for some individuals, they can also have anti-inflammatory properties in others.

People who have gouty inflammatory symptoms may discover that skimmed and low-fat milk is beneficial to their condition.

An elimination diet may help patients identify whether dairy consumption improves or worsens their symptoms.

3. Vegetables from the nightshade family induce inflammation.

Tomatoes, potatoes, eggplants, and peppers all contain solanine, which some attribute to arthritic pain. The Arthritis Foundation, on the other hand, claims that there is no scientific proof supporting this. Including these healthy veggies in your diet may help with a variety of chronic health concerns.

There is evidence that certain meals and minerals may help with osteoarthritis symptoms. They do this by combating inflammation, supplying nutrients, and enhancing bone, muscle, and immune system function.

People may benefit from avoiding or limiting foods that cause inflammation.

Being overweight or obese puts additional strain on the joints, exacerbating the symptoms of osteoarthritis.

People with osteoarthritis may maintain a healthy weight by eating a balanced diet rich in vegetables, fiber, and anti-inflammatory lipids, such as those found in the Mediterranean diet.

This will assist in alleviating symptoms like pain and edema.

How dietary adjustments without calorie limits may aid in healthy aging

Yeast gives scientists a cellular framework in which to test anti-aging drugs and observe their biological reactions.

Short-term diets, according to experts, do not work as well as converting to healthier foods.

They claim that dietary adjustments, rather than calorie restriction, extend life and enhance aging health.

Dietary galactose and calories

Galactose is a simple sugar that, before being utilized as energy, is converted into glucose in the liver. It is common and plentiful in human diets.

According to the International Dairy Federation, galactose is formed from the breakdown of lactose. As a result, dairy products are the most prevalent items in the human diet that contribute to galactose formation.

Fruits, vegetables, nuts, cereals, fresh meat, and eggs are also high in galactose. However, some meals contain just a trace quantity. Milk and yogurt are the principal sources of galactose in the human diet.

The researchers discovered two distinct aging trajectories in budding yeast. When compared to yeast cells that were subjected to intermittent diets, changing the overall type of nutrient intake led to a better aging trajectory.

They imply that a healthy aging trajectory may be feasible depending on the foods you consume. Healthy meals will put you on a healthy path.

Calorie restriction vs. dietary modifications

Weight reduction often entails caloric restriction, which is reducing how much you eat and how many calories you consume each day.

The new research, which used yeast, reveals that changing what you eat rather than how much you consume is healthier and promotes a longer life.

According to the experts, tracking calories is pointless, and eating nutritious meals actually enhances lifespan.

Heart health: How a fruit and veggie prescription might assist
Produce prescriptions allow physicians to write prescriptions for subsidized fresh fruits and vegetables.
A study of produce prescription programs found that participants ate more fruits and vegetables and had lower BMI, blood sugar, and blood pressure.
Food insecurity, which is linked to poor health outcomes, was also decreased by producing prescriptions.
A doctor's prescription for fruits and vegetables may be useful for persons at risk of cardiovascular disease.

Researchers discovered that participants who got a "produce prescription" for six months lowered their body mass index, blood sugar, and blood pressure levels, as well as increased their intake of fruits and vegetables.

Advantages of a Produce Prescription

The individuals in the program were 60% more likely to improve their health condition by one level (for example, from fair to good) at the conclusion of the program, according to the study. Children were twice as likely as adults to report greater health.

Adults who participated in the program improved their consumption of vegetables and fruits by about one cup per day.

Participants with high blood pressure saw their blood pressure drop, while those with diabetes had their blood sugar drop.

The researchers discovered that those with obesity had substantial changes in their body mass index.

Participants were one-third less likely to report food insecurity at the end of the program.

The Effects of Food Insecurity on Health

Food insecurity is defined as a lack of access to or cost of nutritious foods.

An estimated 13.8 million trusted Source families in the United States experienced food insecurity at some time throughout the year in 2020.

More than half of the families in the latest research reported experiencing food insecurity.

According to research, food instability is linked to an elevated risk of cardiovascular disease.

A heart-healthy diet

The American Heart Association Reliable Source recommends consuming a diet high in fruits and vegetables, as well as whole grains.

A healthy protein source, such as nuts, fish, or lean meats, should be included in a well-balanced diet. It is also vital to limit your consumption of added sugar, processed foods, and salt.

Poor eating is the primary cause of sickness in the United States, accounting for more than 500,000 deaths per year. On average, poor eating is responsible for more than 40,000 fatalities per month.